The information contained in this book is intended to be educational and not for diagnosis, prescription, or treatment of any health disorder whatsoever. This information should not replace consultation with a competent healthcare professional.

An important concept I refer to throughout **Girl Lost** is the process of separating the eating disorder from the person. An adolescent or young adult is not her eating disorder. In Chapter Three I talk about this in more detail.

I want to give credit to Thom Rutledge (co-author of Life Without ED and author of Embracing Fear), and James Lock and Daniel Le Grange (authors of Help Your Teenager Beat an Eating Disorder) for this concept.

Their treatment and research contributions are transforming the way we treat adolescents with eating disorders. These ideas have certainly transformed the way I approach adolescent treatment.

I have also done my best to discuss different types of therapy available which includes individual therapy and is still the most common treatment. I have also introduced the more recent form of therapy which is called the Maudsley Approach or Family-Based Treatment.

Girl Lost:

Finding Your Voice through Eating Disorder Recovery

By

By Lynn Moore, MA, LMHC

Note from the Author

How to use this book: **Girl Lost**, a book revealing basic eating disorder information, offers sequentially written ideas regarding the topic. However, you may choose to read the topics and subtopics in any order.

The chapters are intentionally short. You can pick the book up and put it down and read at your own pace. This is not a workbook; though there are a few exercises I encourage you to do because I believe they will help you.

The purpose of this book is to give you basic information about eating disorders. Also to give you an idea of what you may experience as you begin to get help.

If you want more help Lynn coaches parents in re-feeding using the Maudsley Approach. She also does parent consultations per request. You may contact her through her website at www.why-my-daughter.com.

There you can sign up for her free e-book called Eating Disorder Basics for Parents. This will take you straight to her, where you can email her if you so desire.

This book is dedicated to Kinsey.

You were my muse as I wrote this book and my inspiration for any writing I do on this subject. May you find the inspiration to make your mark in the world of writing.

Table of Contents

Girl Lost

By Lynn Moore, MA, LMHC

Chapter 1

One-Sided Conversation

If someone has handed you this small book and asked you to read it, chances are you hear a battle going on in your mind about food. And whomever gave it to you is concerned.

There is a constant conversation in your mind that few know about. It keeps you preoccupied most of your waking hours, often even intruding into your dreams.

And this "conversation" is one-sided. The voice inside your head talks to you. You listen and obey its demands. Some of the statements you have heard so often are now ones you say to yourself.

The conversations may sound something like this:

"I can't eat that. It will make me fat."

"That has too much fat in it."

1

One-Sided Conversation

"I don't know what's in that, so I can't eat it."

"You fat, ugly pig! How could you eat that?"

"You are so weak! You should never have eaten that."

"I don't need food. If I just chew some gum, I won't feel hungry."

"I have to weigh myself."

"That guy looked at me weird. He must think I'm fat!"

"If I can just move the food around on my plate, it will look like I ate more."

"I hate my parents for forcing me to eat."

"I wish I looked like that girl. I'm fat, ugly, and worthless."

"I'll never feel happy."

"Now that I ate that, I have to throw up."

"Now that I ate that, I have to run an extra mile."

"Since I ate that, I can't have breakfast or lunch tomorrow."

"I feel so out of control when I eat."

"I feel afraid to eat."

"I refuse to eat more calories."

"I feel strong when I don't eat."

"I feel powerful when I don't eat."

"I feel empty when I don't eat… and that feels good."

"When I eat, I feel like a failure and hate myself."

"How can I get to a bathroom and get rid of this?"

"What am I going to eat when I get home? Who will be home?"

"What is in the pantry that I can eat? Did Mom buy ice cream last night?"

"My friends can eat anything they want and they don't get fat. Why can't I be like that?"

"I feel so uncomfortable eating in front of other people. I avoid it if at all possible."

"I *did* eat: I had an apple, some grapes, and cereal without milk today."

"I can't stop myself from eating this. I am such a pig. I have no self-control."

"If I eat this, what food can I skip later?"

"I don't need to eat supper anyway. I'll just say I ate before I got home."

"I can't eat what Mom made; it has way too much fat in it."

"I can have half an English muffin but no butter."

"Now that everyone's in bed I can do my crunches."

"I ate that donut, so I might as well eat more. I blew it, so who cares?"

"I hate myself. I hate my body. I hate my thighs. I have a big butt. My arms look too big."

"I hate my stomach; it isn't flat enough."

"Now that I ate, I feel sick to my stomach. I don't feel good. I feel bloated."

"I'd rather be anything than fat."

"I'd rather die than look fat."

"If I can just lose 10 more pounds, then I'll stop. I'll look thin enough."

"I went all day without eating; today was a good day."

"I ate a cookie when I got home; my day is ruined."

"I feel so tired."

"I feel cold all the time."

"When I get rid of what I ate, I feel clean and empty. I like feeling that feeling."

"I can't believe I ate all that. I am such a pig. Once I start, I feel like I can't stop."

If you suffer from an eating issue these are only some of the thoughts that may be going on in your head. There are hundreds if not thousands of ideas that run through your mind in a day.

Your thoughts may be less intense than these examples, or they may be more intense. You may feel obsessed and distracted all the time, or your thoughts may bother you more at certain times of day.

Every person is unique in her thoughts about food, weight, and body. There are, however, similarities that many have in common.

My goal is not to put your thoughts or your behaviors in a box or a category. It is only to help you be more aware of what you think about and how much these thoughts rule your life.

Quick Assignments

~ I want you to stop right now and write down what you are thinking. Just take any sheet of paper, journal and notebook.

Write it all: the good, the bad, the angry, the scared, all of it. This is just for you. No one else has to ever see it. Please don't go on reading until you do this. Do it now.

* * * * *

~ Now I want you to write down any thoughts you have that are food or eating related. You can use ones I mentioned already in this book, and then also write the ones that are unique to you. You have thoughts that are unique to you and your own relationship with the eating disorder.

Write down the thoughts that harass you the most. Again, don't go on reading yet. Go ahead...please write them down. This is for your eyes only unless you choose to share it with someone. Do it now.

* * * * *

Okay, excellent job. I want to tell you that, if you have gone this far, you know there are some thoughts that are causing you pain. These thoughts are like pesky flies that just won't leave you alone. You swat at them repeatedly and they just keep buzzing around you; you can't kill them.

I also want you to know that you are a brave person. You have strength you don't even know about yet.

The thoughts plaguing you and making you behave in confusing ways about food is not easy stuff to admit, think about, or talk about. Most likely you would rather be doing other things instead of the exercises I've asked you do to.

Yet, here you are reading and doing what I asked you to do. Even if there is only a tiny part of you that is willing to do the exercises, to express and reveal your inner most thoughts about your relationship with food...you are listening to that tiny part at this moment. Good for you.

I respect your willingness to even consider that this eating and food stuff may be bigger than you realize. Maybe some of this is out of your control. Maybe you need to hear from someone besides the voice inside your own head.

If you have gotten this far, you must have questions and feel some fear. I want to encourage you to turn the page and keep reading. I will try to be brief and give you only what I think you need to know right now.

I promise not to overwhelm you with information. I just want you to hear that there may be another side to all that is going on in your mind.

Is it possible that the thoughts in your head are not true? That you are being lied to inside your own mind and you don't realize it?

Chapter 2

I Get It!

You may be curious about me, or you may not care. I will be brief, but thought I should at least introduce myself so you know a little about who is talking with you.

I am a therapist and parent coach. I have been working with adolescents, young women and their families who suffer with disordered eating for over 10 years. I have been counseling people for a total of 25 years. So I've been around the block a few times with many who suffer.

I started working with girls with eating issues because I had a 17-year-old client come into my office 10 years ago with anorexia. There was no one else in the area to help her.

I liked her immediately. I enjoy working with women who have eating issues. You are the smartest, brightest, funniest, most caring young women I have ever worked with, and my life has changed because of you.

That may sound weird, but it is true. You have a special place in my heart because I too struggled with fears of getting fat when I was growing up. My mom always battled her weight and my dad often put her down for it.

When my dad said hurtful, critical, condescending opinions about my mother's food and weight issues to Mom, I felt brokenhearted.

But, more importantly, his comments convinced me there was nothing worse than being fat. I grew up falsely believing that gaining weight was to be avoided at all costs.

If I gained weight, I imagined that I would hear words that put me down, rejected, and ridiculed me. Gaining weight was like a fate worse than death.

Meals were stressful because I sat right across the table from my dad and right beside my mom. When my dad would make a comment about my mom's weight, it was like a wall went up between all of us.

There was usually complete silence with hurt and anger hanging in the air like a thick fog. We all knew it was there but acted like nothing had happened. I guess I shouldn't speak for my brothers; I knew the hurt and anger was there.

It was horrible every time. So my mission in life became never to be overweight like my mom. No one was ever going to say those things to me!

The other thing that happened at meal times was that my dad always commented on how little I ate. If I had a dime

I Get It!

for every time he said to me, "You eat like a bird!" I would be rich!

When others said those kinds of remarks to me, I imagined the words reinforced that I was on the right path. I inadvertently trained myself to think, "Eat less, you get positive attention. Eat more, you get shamed and abused."

I lived a long time striving to be the thinnest girl in the room. My identity came from wearing the smallest sizes possible and hearing people comment on how I ate and how I looked.

So I can relate to the thoughts and conversations that go on in your head because I thought them, too. They are punishing and relentless.

Okay, enough about me. Let's get back to you.

Chapter 3

Hearing Voices?

The first thing I want you to consider is that the voice you are hearing in your head is not your own.

What do I mean by that? Don't worry; you do not have multiple personalities. You're not hallucinating, delusional, or crazy.

Many will say that what you're hearing in your head is the voice of an eating disorder. That voice is often called ED, for "eating disorder."

Some call the eating disorder ANA for anorexia; others use the title MIA for bulimia. A few girls come up with a totally different name they are more comfortable with. One girl gave him the name Enemy.

There are two purposes for giving him a name.

1)   It shows that ED is not you, that you are not your eating disorder. If you can see that ED is separate from your own voice, you can be more objective.

When this voice has a name, it is easier for you to consider the possibility that the words you are hearing are coming from someone else. If the words are coming from someone else, they may be easier to evaluate.

2) The fact that ED has a name also makes it easier for us to talk about. It gives us a common language so that, when someone says the word ED, we both know what that means. Some girls don't like the word ED, some prefer it. I will call him ED, because that's what most people are familiar with.

It doesn't really matter what you call him or her. The important thing is to consider the possibility that ED is not you, and there is a possibility that he is not telling you the truth; that he is lying to you.

Just because someone says something to us doesn't automatically mean it is true. It is up to us to hear, evaluate, and either accept or reject the information.

This is true about everything we hear and are told throughout life. It is up to each of us to test the truth of what we are told, no matter who is doing the telling.

I believe ED is actually the voice of your fear.

Your fear of:

- rejection
- not fitting in
- not being good enough
- not being smart enough
- not being pretty enough

- all the hurt you feel in relationships

- your future

Often girls don't even know they have all these fears. All they know is they fear certain foods, gaining weight, and getting fat. All their fears get wrapped up into one box...fear of fat.

It's a lot safer to think about how many calories are in that yogurt, than to admit that you let your friend down and she is mad at you. It's easier to obsess over a number on a scale than it is to think about never being good enough.

It is less painful in some ways to have a list of forbidden foods than it is to deal with how worthless and powerless you actually feel. ED seems to be your pain protection with which you may not know how to cope.

Even as I write this I am thinking yes, in many ways ED is harmful. He tells you all kinds of horrible things about yourself.

But he is also helpful. He shows us there may be a lot of fear in your heart and mind that you didn't even realize was there.

So let's say you are willing to consider the possibility that what you are hearing inside your head is not actually you talking. What you are hearing may not be the truth.

Hearing Voices?

What now? Nothing; I just want you to consider the possibility. That is all I am asking for right now. Oh, and to keep reading.

Chapter 4

Perfectionism

I have met so many adolescent girls who are totally stressed out. Most are so busy with school, sports, music, dance, debate, show choir, friends, homework, and more they don't know how to manage it all.

If you are a young woman in college the pressures may feel intense. You want to get top grades; you may now be a little fish in a big pond where there is more competition. That doesn't include the potential for eating issues in the freshman dorm or living on your own for the first time.

If you are still a teenager you have similar stressors. The primary difference is you have the immediate presence and support of your parents.

The struggle to cope with stress is a huge contributor to the development of eating disorders. The need to perform well and perfectionism are epidemic in our society today.

My guess is that you feel afraid you will fail to perform well enough to please people important to you. Sometimes this expectation comes from high-achieving parents and family. At times it comes mainly from within you. Often it's a combination of both.

Perfectionism

You may look at your mom, dad, or siblings who have achieved much in life. You may believe they expect the same of you, whether they actually do or not. Most girls don't realize their parents only want them to do the best they can.

When I talk with parents and girls about perfectionism, often the parents will smile and say, "She gets that from us." They acknowledge their struggle with perfectionism, too.

We have an open discussion about this issue and she may realize she has internalized this false need to perform. She may begin to see she feels a lot of anxiety because of this.

You may feel some of that, too. You are not alone. You are not the only one who feels the way you do.

Chapter 5

Relationships

Relationships can be very difficult, especially in adolescence and young adulthood. There is often drama with girlfriends that causes an emotional roller coaster inside.

One day you have a best friend; the next day, she has snubbed you and become best friends with someone else. You may not even know why.

For some reason, girls often gravitate toward small groups of three. What happens is one of you always feels left out. The situation is actually a set-up for that to happen.

Threes just don't work well when it comes to friendship. This can cause a lot of hurt and resentful feelings.

Feelings about boys and young men are another land mine. How many times have I heard a girl say, "Why does the guy I like never like me back?" The desire to be loved and accepted for who you are by someone can feel all-consuming.

It's very emotionally painful to watch other girls have what you desire. Often you decide there must be something wrong with you.

The error many make is to simplify it all down to one belief or perception. You don't have what you desire because you are fat, and the solution to this problem is to lose weight.

What starts as a simple diet turns into something you never anticipated. Most girls don't wake up one morning and say, "I think I will develop an eating disorder." It just doesn't happen that way.

The other relationship that can cause stress is with your family. Most likely you can point to areas of frustration and conflict between you and your parents; or between you and your siblings (what kid can't). How many families do you know who don't have any problems or conflicts?

In the family where someone has an eating disorder, conflict may be part of the family relationships. The goal is to learn to communicate and negotiate problems.

This doesn't mean you're eating disorder is your parent's or family's fault. I am just pointing out that family relationships can cause stress and stress can contribute to the development and maintenance of ED.

So here is what can happen: Parents, guys, and girlfriends let you down; ED won't. Human relationships result in disappointment and hurt. ED is always there when you need him, because he is the voice inside your mind.

People will reject and leave you; ED won't. He is always there. ED and food become your primary relationships because they are your safety net.

Your life revolves increasingly around food. What you can and can't eat; what you did eat and how you have to compensate for it; how many miles you have to run; how often you have to go to the gym. Your world shrinks to only food-related thoughts and feelings.

So one of the things you have to do is to change your relationship with ED and food. You have to become re-connected with life and the people you love.

You have temporarily forgotten: there's a whole world out there with fun people, exciting things to do, passions to pursue, and a LIFE! ED has convinced you he is your life.

The reality is that ED is trying to take your life from you. The people who love you are trying to help you get it back. I encourage you to give someone besides ED a chance. ED may be lying to you. I believe he is.

Chapter 6

I Don't Want to Go!

There is the possibility that if you are reading this book, someone wants you to go to counseling. My guess is you don't want to go and would do almost anything to avoid going to counseling.

Now, some of you might actually be relieved that your parents are asking you to do this, or you may have even asked for it yourself. Many of you, though, do not want to get help.

Can I just say I don't blame you? That may sound silly, coming from a therapist.

But seriously, who *does* want to go sit in some stranger's office and spill her guts? Some do but my experience is most people do not; myself included. I have had my share of counselors over the years and I know it is not easy.

Here is how one of my young clients described her first session in counseling:

"I've always been awkward and rather uncomfortable going to meet new people when it's not my decision to do so, and it was no different when I met my therapist...at first. I went in for the first time with both of my parents.

"I remember sitting on the tan couch feeling like a shell. My skin was just a layer, and beneath it, all I had were thoughts. Loads of them; but it was impossible to listen or recognize them all.

"One thing I distinctly remember about the first session was she went over why I was there having the session to begin with. I remember hearing the words 'eating disorder' just hanging in the air, and all I wanted to do was hide and cry; I only managed to do the latter.

"But in a way, it was a relief and my shell could breathe again. And every time I went back it was as if I could slowly take bigger and deeper breaths."

There are pros and cons to talking to a counselor. I want to talk to you about both. Let's start with the cons, because that may be what you're thinking about most right now.

Cons:

- You may not like talking to adults, especially ones you don't know

- The expectation is for you to talk about things you don't even understand yourself, let alone say out loud to someone else

- You may feel scared and uncomfortable

- You might feel angry with your parents and not want to talk about it with them

- You may feel you don't have a problem, that your parents are blowing this way out of proportion, and that it's all a waste of time

- You may think this whole thing is stupid

- You might have to talk about some things that make you uncomfortable

- You may feel stupid, embarrassed, and ashamed

- You may have no clue what to say

- You might feel afraid to feel your true feelings

- Or maybe you just want to do something else with that hour

Pros:

- Your parents will calm down

- As much as you may not want to admit this, it might help to have an objective person help you figure all this out

- There are very few people who really listen to you, and how often do you get someone who will listen for an hour straight and focus *completely* on how you feel and what you think?

- There are times when you probably do feel out of control and overwhelmed; talking to someone may help you feel less stressed out and overwhelmed

- You may feel depressed at times and it might help to have a place to go with all the negative thoughts, feelings and mind images about yourself, your body, your friends and family

- You might someday be able to live without the constant running commentary in your head about food, body, and a number on a scale

- You could go hang out with friends again and have a silly piece of pizza and feel normal like everyone else

- Maybe you could even sleep over at a friend's house and not demand that your mom pick you up before they all eat pancakes

- You might be able to eat without throwing it up and not have to worry about being caught

- Perhaps you could exercise or run cross-country because you enjoy it, not because you have to get rid of the calories you ate today

- Maybe you could eventually sit down at the dinner table with your family and not have World War III

I Don't Want to Go!

- Your phone conversations with your parents might be less stressful if they knew you were getting help

I have not purposefully come up with more pros than cons to try and make it look better than it is. You can probably come up with some cons I didn't think about.

You might even come up with a few more pros, I don't know. I just wanted to give you an idea of what writing pros and cons might look like, and what some of them could be.

Sometimes girls are told to choose between coming to see me for counseling or going into hospital in-patient treatment. Needless to say, most choose me, but that doesn't mean they are thrilled about it.

You may not be thrilled either but I'd encourage you to give it a try. It just might help.

Chapter 7

Do I Have to Lie on the Couch?

So let's say you decide to give this counseling thing a try. What will happen when you get there?

Don't worry. I don't know any counselors who ask clients to lie down on the couch anymore. Thank goodness!

One or both of your parents will most likely talk to a receptionist and discuss the financial aspects of all this. They will talk about insurance and schedule appointments.

If you're in college your appointment may be at the college counseling center. You may continue to be seen there or they may refer you to someone in the community who ideally specializes in eating disorders.

The office will probably be similar to a doctor's office, but may be more nicely furnished. Most counseling offices feel a bit homey, in the hope that you will feel more comfortable.

There will be a waiting room and probably a few other people waiting to see their counselors. This may feel a bit weird, and you may feel exposed and embarrassed at first. Many girls want to be invisible at this point.

25

While you wait, you can listen to your iPod or text your friends. Hopefully you won't have to wait long. Some bring books to read or do homework.

Sometimes counselors get behind, just like doctors. They won't just kick people out of their office when the hour is up. How insensitive would that be? "Sorry, I know you're sitting here crying, but our time is up, so you've got to go."

I try really hard to stay on time and most therapists do. If she does run late, just remember: there may come a day when you need that extra few minutes, and you'll be glad you waited patiently when others needed it.

When your counselor is ready, she will open a door somewhere and call your name. You may look at your parents at the last second with an expression that implies, "Do I *really* have to do this?"

They will nod their heads *yes*. They may give you a *look* you've seen before, and then you and/or your parents will get up and follow the counselor into the office.

Most likely the counselor will ask you and your parents "What brings you in today?" or something else very professional and adult-like. Either your mom or your dad will probably start. Often moms talk first.

Your parents will explain why you are there and what has been going on. Eventually you will be asked why you think you are there and what your thoughts and feelings are about all this.

Some counselors will treat it more like an interview. They will ask direct questions like, "How many calories are you getting in a day? What do you typically eat for breakfast?"

Some may focus on basic education and explain some of the things I have told you. They will try to give you an overview of what is going to happen.

Others will be more laid back. They may ask some questions just to get to know you; like the things you do for fun and what your interests are.

They may ask who your friends are and what you all do together, stuff like that. Most therapists will probably do a combination of all the above.

Here is what I want you to know. You are probably initially going to feel emotionally uncomfortable. You will, however, be able to tell if this counselor is someone you believe is "getting" what you are saying.

You will feel like she is listening to you and cares about you. You may not have that feeling with every therapist, and it is okay to tell your parents your opinions about the therapist when you leave. It is okay to ask to see a different counselor next time.

One caution is worth mentioning here. A part of you may want to reject *any* counselor because you don't want to do this whole "counseling thing." But I want you to remember the pros and cons and what you can gain from this person.

If you feel like this therapist gets what you are saying, listens to you, and seems to care about you, I would really encourage you to go back. Give her a chance to help.

* * * * *

Let me tell you something about counselors and therapists. Very few of us do what we do for the money.

It is understandable for you to think that we are listening because we are being paid to do it. Many think we are being paid to care, so our desire to help is dismissed. I hear that a lot, actually.

The reality is that there is no amount of money that would make it worthwhile to me to sit in a room all day with people in pain. It's not easy to sit, hour after hour, and listen to people pour out their deepest hurts and fears.

I do it *because* I care, not because I get paid for it. Most of us would not pursue this kind of work if we didn't care, because we would never last. It's just too hard.

Besides, we don't get paid *that* much. I could do something else where I would get paid a lot more. But I choose to sit in a room with you because I *do* care and I *do* want to help.

I just want to help you understand the person you are going to sit across from and talk with. She cares deeply, or she wouldn't be there. The counselor wants to get to know you and hear from you; she wants to help you.

So let me speak for myself and other therapists out there. We are truly here for you, if you want us.

If you don't, that's something you have to figure out with your parents. We care, we will listen, and we will do everything within our power to help.

* * * * *

Let's get back to what therapy is like. Usually after the first appointment with you and your parents, your counselor will want to meet with you alone. At times a counselor will meet first with you; it really just depends.

She will then probably ask to meet with your parents alone. At some point she may want to see the whole family, siblings included, because everyone is impacted by ED.

If you are in college the counselor may ask if she can call your parents or doctor. I'll say more about this later.

You will probably meet weekly for a period of time. Your parents and siblings will be involved here and there.

Now, I know you may be thinking, "Why is this all about me? My family has problems, too." This may be true, and hopefully in this process, all of you will get help.

I do want to give you a heads up because things are changing in the counseling world when it comes to dealing with eating disorders. The focus is turning more toward the family and less on you, the individual.

There are more therapists who are starting to deal almost exclusively with the family as a whole. Every session may involve the family.

Again, if you are in college you may be too far away for much parent and family involvement. It just depends on your circumstances.

Some therapists may ask your parents to bring a meal to the session and the family will eat it with the therapist present. Yeah, I know; this may seem like a scary and frustrating idea.

The purpose of family based treatment is for your parents to learn how to help you eat more even when it is difficult for you. Your parents will be coached how to feed you at home. This type of family work; also called the Maudsley Approach will continue throughout the process of helping you eat at home.

With this approach any individual issues you may have like perfectionism or depression will not be addressed until you are at a healthy weight. Many young women find their depression and anxiety decrease as they gain weight. Some do not need individual therapy at all.

As I mentioned, family involvement and parent re-feeding is a change that is occurring in the treatment of eating disorders. It is however, happening slowly, as change often does.

I wouldn't be surprised if your counselor makes changes over time in how he or she tries to help. Be as open and as flexible to the ideas of change as you can because, just like in medicine, the world of computers, the automobile industry, new things are being discovered all the time.

My guess is, just for right now though, after the first few sessions, the therapist will focus on you because that is still the most common form of treatment. As I said, please consider being open to the therapy ideas your counselor suggests.

The goal in individual counseling is for you to develop a trusting and safe relationship with your counselor. We want you to say pretty much anything you want or need to without fear of judgment or criticism.

All of us need someone in our lives we can be totally honest with...who knows the good and the bad and still loves us. For this time in your life, one of those people can be your counselor.

You have a lot going on, and friends aren't always the best ones to rely on for counsel. They can support you and listen, but most of them may be experiencing some of the same things you are. It may be difficult for them to act truly objective with you.

Plus, they may feel afraid of hurting your feelings or losing your friendship. Their need for your friendship may hinder their ability to act totally honest with you.

Do you know that it's often a friend who actually reveals the secret of your eating issues? This true friend will usually go to her (sometimes his) parents and tell them what is going on with you.

If she knows your parents well enough, she may even tell your parents herself. It may feel scary for friends to act and speak that honestly. No one wants to lose a friend, and if she tells your secret she knows you may not like what she did and may not like to be her friend anymore.

Your counselor will always be honest with you and have your best interest in mind. As you come to believe you can trust your counselor more, you will choose to talk about more of your ideas and feelings. Talking often will help you begin to feel better.

You will feel less depressed or less anxious. As you express your ideas and feelings, you will learn how to cope with stress better and how to handle difficult relationships and feelings.

You will hopefully start to feel more like your old self again and may even hear your parents say something like, "I feel like I am getting my daughter back." Most likely you will begin to see that you were more obsessed by food, calories, weight, and your body than you even realized.

Things will start to make sense again and you won't feel as confused and scared. You will be able to make a mistake or have a disagreement with a friend and it won't feel like the end of the world.

The combination of weight restoration and counseling if necessary will help you get better. Ideally we want you to be able to eat anything, anywhere at any time and not feel anxious or depressed.

Eventually no foods will be frightening or forbidden. It will only be necessary to sustain life and at times to enjoy in moderation. Food is your medicine so you can get well; that is its only purpose.

Chapter 8

What Is a Treatment Team?

One of the phrases you will most likely hear is "treatment team." This means that along with your therapist, there will probably be a physician and perhaps a nutritionist.

I think the physician's role is pretty obvious. He or she will do blood work, and an overall health exam. He or she does all of this so he or she can have a baseline of your body's chemistry and monitor your health.

The physician will look for possible side effects from your eating behaviors or lack thereof. You will hear the doctor's opinion about the diagnosis of an eating disorder and his or her recommendations.

The doctor may recommend in-patient treatment which means hospitalization if your health is at risk. Or you may be referred to a local therapist and a nutritionist.

You may be prescribed medication that could help with depression or anxiety. This is totally dependent upon your physician, you, and your parents. You and your parents decide if medication is right for you.

The nutritionist's role is to help you figure out a healthy amount of food to eat. Often with eating disorders, girls and women forget what is normal. They don't know what too much or too little food is.

The nutritionist may come up with a food menu for you along with your input. You may also be asked to keep a food journal of what you eat each day. Every nutritionist is different, so these recommendations may vary.

A nutritionist may also help you understand so you can decide an appropriate amount of exercise for you to do. Sometimes you forget what a healthy amount of exercise is, just like you do with food.

Knowing a healthy amount of exercise is especially important if exercise is one of the ways you try to get rid of what you eat. If you are over-taxing your body with too few calories or purging, exercise will probably be limited.

I want to give you a heads-up here about nutritionists. She has the toughest job of all of us who are trying to help.

Why? A nutritionist has to talk with you directly about food and perhaps about adding food into your daily meal plan; unless you are involved in Family Based Treatment (FBT). With FBT your parents will make the primary food decisions.

You will most likely *not* be thrilled to have food added to your meal plan. It will be tempting for you to take your anger out on your nutritionist.

And on your parents as they become more insistent about what, when and how much you eat. The nutritionist and your parents can even begin to feel like an enemy to you and ED.

Remember to consider that the voice you've named ED may say things that misrepresent himself and his motives, especially about those professionals who are intending to help you. ED may suggest the professionals and your parents are the bad guys when they are actually the good guys.

My encouragement to you is: be as honest and direct with your anger as possible. Remember that a lot of your anger is probably anxiety about having to eat more.

Tell your therapist and your parents about these feelings. If you can tell the nutritionist too, that would be great. She can help with your anxiety also.

I also encourage you to keep going to your nutritionist. It is pretty common for young women to stop these appointments because of anxiety. I'm going to say a bit more about going to appointments in Chapter 10.

Hang in there and let your nutritionist be a part of helping you get better. Your nutritionist's role in helping you re-learn about food is important.

You and your parents are also on your "treatment team." It is important for you to know you have a voice in your treatment and recovery; as do your parents if you are under age.

I will talk more about the importance of your voice in a bit. I just want you to understand the different people who may be intending to help.

Chapter 9

My Parents Are Driving Me Crazy!

Let me tell you something about parents. They have heard horror stories about girls dying from eating disorders. How parents pay thousands of dollars for treatment for their daughters; and often the treatment doesn't help. How families are torn to shreds because a child has an eating disorder.

Your parents feel scared. And when parents feel scared, they say and do things they wouldn't ordinarily say and do. Or maybe they would say it, but this is much more intense.

Your mom is afraid that, if she can't get you to eat or stop throwing up, you will die. Let's face it, some people die. Go to www.somethingfishy.com and click on the Memorial tab.

There is a candle and person's name for every death from an eating disorder. And these are just the ones that get reported to this site. Your parents want to avoid adding your name to this website.

Another terrible thing parents hear is how someone's daughter never got help. She is now an adult, still struggling with eating issues.

She is still starving herself or throwing up 20 years later. That terrifies your parents. They feel afraid this will happen to you.

So one of the things I encourage you to do is go easy on your parents. I know that may sound crazy or even unfair.

After all, *you* are the one struggling with this eating disorder; why can't they get it together and calm down? They can't because they love you too much.

When you agree to talk with someone or begin FBT, your parents may start to calm down. It still won't be all butterflies and rainbows with them, but it can be *better*.

They will feel relieved that someone knows what to do and how to help, because your parents often don't realize they have the strength to do what is best. And that is to help you eat more. This eating disorder is new to them, too.

They are not used to you being sullen, irritable, or angry. The daughter they know didn't used to fight at dinner about food, or yell at them on the phone. You were probably the low-maintenance kid before all this happened.

Most likely you acted very social, outgoing, and funny. You wanted to be with friends, and still wanted to be part of the family.

You probably enjoyed going out for pizza with the family on a Friday night, and couldn't wait to go out with friends. They have seen changes in you and they don't understand why or how to get you back.

So, if you can, imagine seeing the situation through their eyes. Think about how this must feel to them. How important it is that they know you are getting what you need to feel better.

Like it or not, whether you admit it out loud or not, if you are reading this book then something is wrong. You are feeling different than you used to feel, and you are feeling some kind of pain either emotional, mental or physical or all three.

Your parents are not stupid, even if it seems like it to you at times. They know you. They recognize change when they see it, and something in you has changed.

The question is whether or not you will admit it. And, as scary as it might feel; are you willing to do something to improve your situation?

Chapter 10

I Have Choices?

I also want to talk to you about the choices you have in all this, because you do have them. You may not feel like you do, but you do.

You may be thinking, "What do you mean, I have a choice? My mom is making me go to these appointments!"

Here is what I mean. You know your parents will not physically pick you up, stuff you in the car kicking and screaming, and drag you into the counseling office.

They will not and cannot hold you down and force food down your throat. Granted, they can hospitalize you without your consent, but they are hoping and praying it will not come to that.

"So what?" you ask. "I still don't feel like I have a choice." Since they cannot physically force you into a counseling office, this means you are making a choice to go to your appointments.

It also means you make the choice to eat at times when you don't want to or don't feel like it. If you decide not to fight, you are making a choice. It may not feel like it is a choice, but it is.

Another choice you have is how open you will be once you get to an appointment. You can sit silently in the therapist's office for an hour, or you can give her a chance to hear your side of the story.

Your parents are certainly going to give their view on the issue. It seems to me you deserve the same opportunity.

If going to therapy has been a huge or small battle between you and your parents, I want to encourage you. Take control of the situation in a healthy way.

Make the decision yourself to go and get what you can out of it. We've already talked about the positive things that could happen as a result.

Many girls feel that, if they "give in" and go to therapy, they lose and their parents win. This is not about someone winning and someone losing.

This is about your life. Not your parents' life, but your life.

And I don't mean that just in a literal way, that eating disorders can kill you (between 5% and 20% die from the disease). I mean that you have your whole life ahead of you and you have a choice about how you are going to live it; within reason of course if you are under age.

- Do you want to continue feeling obsessed by thoughts about food all day long, or do you prefer to develop a healthier relationship with food and eating.

- When you go out with your friends now or in college, do you want to sit and envy them for being able to eat freely, or do you want to be a part of the group?

- If you have been starving yourself, do you want to continue to feel cold all the time, weak and even faint, or do you want to be able to play basketball, volleyball, or run track with the strength you had in the past?

- Do you want to continue to be in pain when you sit in your chair at school because of bone on wood, or do you want to feel comfortable and free of pain?

- If you have been throwing up the food you eat, do you want to continue to feel the anxiety and urgency to get to the bathroom after you eat? Do you always want to worry about being discovered purging, or do you want to stay at the table with your friends and have fun?

- Do you want to continue to feel shame and worthlessness after purging or a sense of achievement and strength because you chose to respect your body by digesting your food instead of throwing it up?

I Have Choices?

This is what I mean by you have a choice. I want you to see that working to understand and change your attitudes about food is not just about whether or not you go to a therapist or nutritionist or doctor appointment.

It is about how you want to spend the rest of your life. How you want to feel, what you want to do, who you want to be with, and who you are going to be as a person.

Will you be a person who uses her intelligence, caring heart, sense of humor, and strength in order to contribute to the world? Or will you get lost forever in this obsession with food, weight, body, and calories?

Are you going to participate fully in your relationships or remain on the outside looking in, longing to eat like your friends eat?

It may feel good to be the smallest girl in the room, but let's face it; you may also be the loneliest. I've been there, and lonely hurts.

So yes, you have a choice. You have a lot of them, actually. The question is; will you realize that you have choices and take healthy control of your life?

Successful people are not successful because they are the thinnest or prettiest. Nor are they happy because they are with an *attractive* person.

They are successful and happy because they take responsibility for their lives and choose their path wisely. They decide what they want and work hard to get it.

What they want is not perfection, but to feel happy with the things they do during their lives. You can be happy too; just make the right choice.

- With ED in control, you lose close relationships with people because you are never really present with them. Part of you is with them, the other part is obsessing about food.

- When ED is running you're life, you give your control over to food, rituals, rules, and a number on the scale, calories, and a task master that will dictate every decision.

- When ED is in charge, you lose the freedom to be a participant in life and become an envious and lonely observer.

- When ED is in control, you subject yourself to constant abuse from ED. He is always there to tell you how you screwed up, are weak, and have no will power. That you are fat, ugly, stupid, and a failure.

- And this verbal abuse is just the tip of the iceberg. ED will never run out of destructive and frightening things to say.

I Have Choices?

I understand that at the beginning you do not feel like you have a choice. It feels like ED is fully in control and that may be true.

If you allow people to help you, that will change and you will increasingly feel like you do have a choice. Until that day comes, you have to trust those who love you and at least start to question ED and his motives.

Chapter 11

ED the Poseur

Let's talk a bit more about ED and who he is. I want you to consider the possibility that ED is not who you think he is.

Right now you may believe that ED is helping you. He is helping you lose weight or at least not gain weight.

You may think he is going to help you get what you want. You may want popularity, success, acceptance, a boyfriend/girlfriend, a whole number of things.

I mean, let's think about it. When you watch television commercials and movies, the happy and successful women are the thin ones; right? The happy guys are the tall, buff, athletic looking ones with the beautiful girl on the beach.

Gorgeous girls lean up against the newest Lexus on the market, walk sensually along the shore with the handsome guy, wear the coolest and most sexy clothes and the best make-up and perfumes. The list is endless.

Who doesn't want all that? If that's happiness, then bring it on; right? This is where ED waltzes into your life and mind. He convinces you he can get you all of that if you just follow his instructions.

Here is the problem: ED's praise and acceptance of you are conditional. If you do what he tells you to do, he praises and encourages you that you are doing the right thing.

If you don't do what he tells you to do, he puts you down, accuses you, even verbally abuses you. He becomes this internal bully who won't let up.

You want someone to love you for who you are, yet ED is just like you feel about everyone else. His acceptance depends upon you doing what he thinks you should do or what he tells you to do.

So in reality he is no different than friends and family who will unintentionally, but inevitably hurt you. The difference is that ED is intentionally hurting you. You just may not know it yet.

You may or may not have thought of this before, but go ahead and test this out. Try disobeying what you hear him say in your mind, and see what happens.

If he says you cannot eat butter on your toast because it will make you fat, try eating butter on your toast and see what thoughts come and what he tells you. I promise you: it will not be pretty.

I want you to consider the possibility that, even though he has convinced you he is here to help you, he may not truly have your best interest in mind. He says he wants to help you lose weight, get friends, be beautiful, and more. Yet how does he treat you?

If you had a boyfriend who said he loved you, but put you down constantly, what would you think? If he told you how fat and ugly you were when you ate or didn't throw up, would you really believe he cared about you?

Or would you think he has another agenda? If you had a girlfriend who was in a relationship with an abusive boy, what would you tell her?

Hopefully, whether it was you or a girlfriend in this situation, you would consider the possibility that he is not who he presents himself to be. I am asking you to do the same thing with ED.

He wants you to think he is for you, and he is: as long as you comply. But disobey him, and watch out!

His acceptance is frighteningly conditional! And you will hear more abuse from him than you will ever hear from your parents or friends. The scary part is you will begin to believe all the bad things he says to you and about you.

Think about who you are listening to most right now? Does he deserve to have that much of a voice and that much power in your decisions?

What about *your* voice? The voice of the young woman you used to be and the woman you are to become. The one who:

- Loved ice cream

- Would never eat a salad without salad dressing; how boring is that?

- Couldn't wait for your mom's lasagna and cheesecake for dessert

- Spent time with friends that included eating your favorite munchies

- Looked forward to birthdays and special occasions without fear of cake

- Ate a reasonable amount of food and didn't have to run to the bathroom

- And on, and on, and on

Your voice has gotten lost because ED's voice is so loud. He is so obnoxious you can't hear anything else. You have to seek your voice again and tell ED to be quiet.

* * * * *

As we wrap up, I want you to take this time to think about who you were before this voice (ED) entered your mind. I would encourage you to write down your answers to these questions.

- What did you used to enjoy doing that you no longer do?

- What were some of your favorite foods that you no longer eat?

- What were things you used to do with friends that you don't do anymore?

- How would you describe yourself before ED came along? (happy, fun, caring)

- How would you describe yourself now? (worried, irritable, lonely)

- What or who do you want to be like now?

- Are you happy with whom you are right now?

- What would your friends say is different about you now versus before?

- What would your brothers or sisters say is different?

- What would your parents say is different?

- What do you want to be doing in 2, 5 or 10 years?

- What role do you want food to play in your life?

- How do you want to think and feel about food?

* * * * *

Now, I want you to go back and read Chapter 10 about choices. It is important. I want you to decide what kind of life you want.

Not what your parents want and certainly not ED! What do *you* want and what are you willing to go through to get it?

You can do this. This may be one of the most important decisions you ever make. Look ED straight in the eye and see him for who he really is.

I want you to consider the possibility that he is an imposter, a *poseur*. He may not be the true friend you think he is.

* * * * *

One last assignment:

I would strongly encourage you to write a letter to your parents after you read this book. A letter will give you the chance to think through what you want to say. It will be less emotional the first time you are trying to put words to your thoughts and feelings.

Tell them what you learned and what you are thinking about. Tell them what you want from them if you know. If you don't know, that is okay too. The purpose is just to get communication going.

A letter will give your parents time to think about what you have written. It will help them approach you with less emotion because they will have had time to deal with their emotions as well.

If you are willing to write a letter, it will make the next conversations much easier. This stuff can be difficult to talk about, and I want to make it as easy on you as possible. Give it a shot. I really think it will help.

I also would encourage you to write a letter to ED. Tell him in the letter how you feel about him, what you want from him and what you want to change in your relationship.

Just be honest with him and yourself. Write it like he is sitting right in front of you and you are telling him what you think and feel. Get it all out. Tell him everything.

If you have a therapist, take the letter with you and share it. Or share it with your parents or another adult you trust. Or not; it is totally up to you.

* * * * *

Here is the bottom line. Look at your life and see the people who really love and care for you. They aren't perfect; they probably have let you down in some ways, but they love you. And they want to help you fight this and get well.

They want to hear your voice again; the voice of their daughter, sister, cousin, granddaughter, niece, friend. Not ED.

Make a choice and just take the first step; whatever that first step is for you. That's all you need to do right now is take one tiny step, whatever it is.

Don't think about it. If you do you will give ED time to talk you out of it.

What is YOUR VOICE telling you to do? Go do it; now. I'm in your corner and so are a lot of other people. Go; do, take action.

Addendum: If You Are in College

If you are in college or out of your parent's home, you have most of the power and your parents have little. What I mean by that is they have little leverage to increase the chances you will get help.

You're not a teenager so most likely they won't take your cell phone or stop paying your bill; they probably won't take your car keys or try to dish out consequences like when you were younger.

Ultimately they could stop paying for college and force you to come home; so I guess they do have that leverage. But they don't want to do that. They want you to be in college and successful in your education and career.

They may try to talk to you about their concerns and all you have to do is shut them down with your anger. You can hang up the phone, tell them not to visit and basically shut them out of your life.

I want you to consider that as soon as they mention anything to do with food, weight or purging, ED steps in and takes over the conversation. It is not you reacting to your parent's legitimate love and concern, it is ED.

ED has convinced you he is the only one who can help you. He seductively persuades you to believe that anyone else, even your parents who you know would never intentionally hurt you, is only trying to make you fat.

Wow...what power ED has. He has the power to:

- take a relationship you have had with your parents for eighteen plus years and destroy it

- make you turn on the very people who have helped you get to where you are today

- turn the person you were into a person you and those who love you don't even know

- influence your thoughts to a point where instead of eating more you might actually die

- rob you of some of the best years of your life and all because of a number on a scale

- push your friends away to the point where you are so lonely you don't want to live anymore

- make you feel so guilty you will never do anything to go against him

- keep you in bondage to food, calories, and weight for a life time

- take away your ability to choose for yourself what to eat, where you can go, who you hang out with, and how to treat people who love you

That's a lot of power. You don't have to lose all that. I know you currently feel afraid of eating more, not bingeing and purging, not over-exercising, and not engaging in eating disorder behaviors.

I really do get that. I just hope you will consider that you can never get the years back that you give to ED and this illness. Some people lose a whole lifetime to a lie and this is the most terrifying of all.

What if what you see, think and feel really is a lie? Are you willing to risk all you've worked for, your relationships and your future for something that might be a lie?

If your parents or others who care about you reach out, give them a chance. Consider that the voice you are hearing in your mind is not the one you should be listening to.

You've trusted your parents before... trust them again. They aren't perfect, they've made mistakes, but they love you more than ED ever could. Besides ED's motives are not to love you; they are to control you.

Acknowledgements

I want to thank first of all my husband Patrick. Without him I would never have had the courage to follow my dreams.

How can I acknowledge those who have helped and inspired me without thanking God? He is my Rock, my Foundation in everything I do, think, feel and believe.

I will always be thankful for each and every client who taught me much of what I know about how to help with eating disorders. Two especially always come to mind; Jennifer and Kinsey.

Each girl I worked with have loving parents and I am honored they trusted me enough to work with them and their wonderful daughters. Those parents are Tom, Denise, Scott and Terry.

There are two other people I would like to mention. It is because of their strong and guiding voices, this book came into being.

Sean Mize and Beverly Taylor have coached me through treacherous waters. They helped me take my love for young women, eating disorders and therapy and transfer it to online coaching.

Finally I wish to thank my family. During the good times and the bad, they have been behind the scenes loving and supporting me.

Thanks also to Cynthia Hilton, Susan Fox my editors and Chantal Lily who provided the book cover design. Your gifts made this process easier than I ever would have imagined.

Many I have not mentioned have been with me in spirit on this project. I believe they know who they are. Thank you.

I hope this book helps young women and their families; and makes it a bit less frightening as you begin this journey to recovery. We all need someone in our corner. I'm in yours.

Lynn Moore

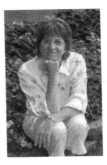

About the Author

Lynn has her Master's degree in Counseling and has been in the counseling field for over 25 years. She is licensed in the State of Iowa as a *Licensed Mental Health Counselor* and has specialized in eating disorders for over 10 years.

She is an *Eating Disorder Parent Coach*, psychotherapist, author and artist. Lynn lives with her husband in Indianola, Iowa in their little brown house in the woods. There her creativity well is filled daily by nature, wildlife and the comfort of home and rural community.

If you want more help Lynn coaches parents in re-feeding using the Maudsley Approach. You may contact her through her website at www.why-my-daughter.com.

There you can sign up for her free e-book called Eating Disorder Basics for Parents. This will take you straight to her, where you can email her if you so desire.

Resources for Young Women

Websites

www.somethingfishy.com

www.eating-disorder-information.com

www.eatingdisorderhope.com

www.pale-reflections.com

www.bulimia.com

Books *Christian Resources

*Beyond STARVED: Real Stories of Real Freedom by Nancy Alcorn Available at www.mercyministries.org - 2009

Goodbye Ed, Hello Me: Recover from Your Eating Disorder and Fall in Love with Life by Jenni Schaefer - 2009

Life Without Ed: How One Woman Declared Her Independence from Her Eating Disorder and How You Can Too by Jenni Schaefer and Thom Rutledge - 2003

*Starved: Mercy for Eating Disorders by Nancy Alcorn Available at www.mercyministries.org – 2007

The Stress Reduction Workbook for Teens by Gina M. Biegel - 2009

Understanding Your Eating Disorder (Teen Tips) by Waln K. Brown - Kindle eBook – 2008

Resources for Parents

Websites

www.feast-ed.org/

www.maudsleyparents.org/faqs.html

Books

Brave Girl Eating by Harriet Brown - 2010

Eating with Your Anorexic by Laura Collins - 2004

Embracing Fear by Thom Rutledge – 2002

Help Your Teenager Beat an Eating Disorder by James Lock and Daniel Le Grange – 2005

Skills-based Learning for Caring for a Love One with an Eating Disorder by Janet Treasure – 2007

*Any resource cited for young women on the previous page would be helpful for any parent to read.

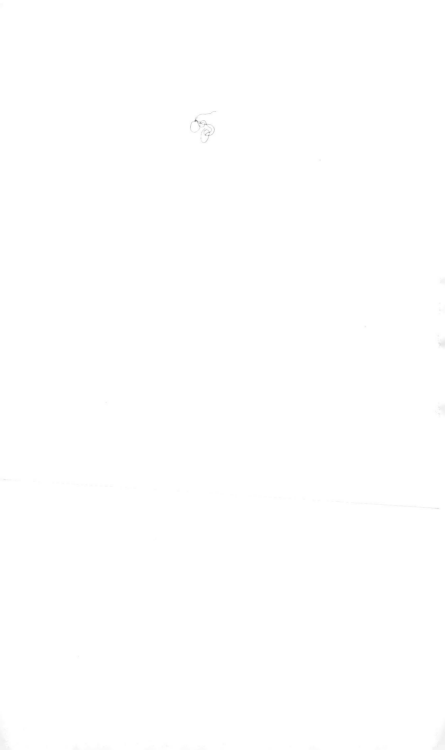

36784323R00040

Made in the USA
Lexington, KY
04 November 2014